EATING YOURSELF THIN

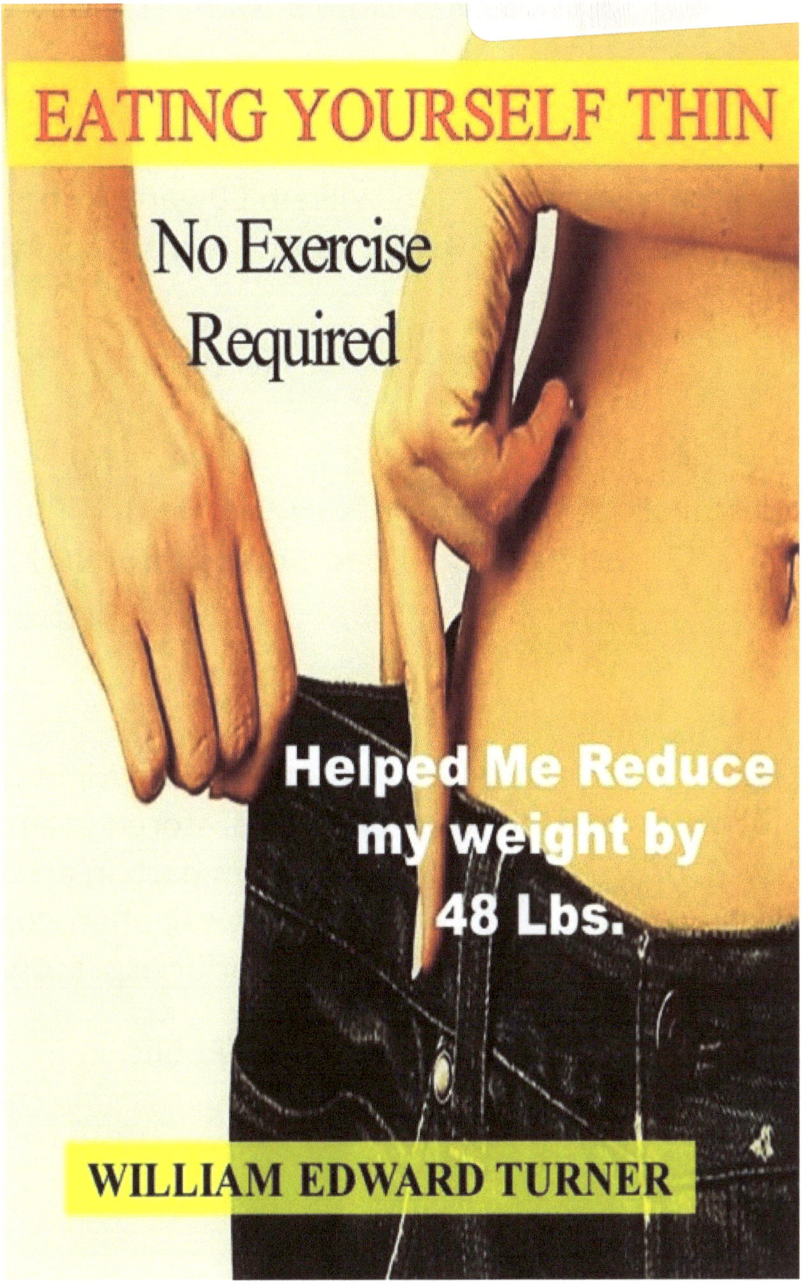

No Exercise Required

Helped Me Reduce my weight by 48 Lbs.

WILLIAM EDWARD TURNER

Eating Yourself Thin

By Minister William Edward Turner

Copyright © 2016 William Edward Turner
Narrow Gate Ministries of Greensboro, Inc.

ISBN: 9781097878628

Narrow Gate Ministries of Greensboro, Inc. Publisher
522-203B College Road Greensboro, NC 27410

Eating Yourself Thin

Eating Yourself Thin Strategy Was created out of my personal need to reduce my weight. After I was hospitalized for about 5 years I had gained 63 pounds. I was unable to exercise and depressed because I could not fit any of my clothes. Nothing I tried worked with lasting results. Plus my medications make me feel like I was starving. I could eat dinner and before I was done I was thinking about what I would eat later. Besides this food had now become my comforting friend.

"I prayed to God show me what to do and He did."

The Eating Yourself Thin Strategy has helped me reduce my weight by 48 pounds. In this book I attempt to be as real as possible. I talk about how others see you and the rude things people say. Eating everything not nailed down. Craving for those goodies I have stopped eating. Problems I had with diets and regaining pounds.

Eating Yourself Thin

This Strategy involves looking at food from a different perspective. You do not have to buy special foods, go to no classes and do no exercises unless you feel like it. Stopping the strategy without weight return whiplash. When you get off track just get back on. Yes it does take discipline but you can do all things through Christ who strengthens you.

Minister William Edward Turner

Eating Yourself Thin

Note: If you are sick and/or under medical care, taking medication(s), have a diagnosed medical condition or disease, pregnant or lactating, younger than 21 – please consult with your physician before using the **Eating Yourself Thin Strategy.** Narrow Gate Ministries of Greensboro, Inc. is not responsible for adverse effects of above mentioned conditions.

.

Eating Yourself Thin

"Eating Yourself Thin" is NOT a Diet

and Exercising is Not Required.

Eating Yourself Thin is about looking at your food intake from a different prospective. The focus is not losing weight or eating only certain foods. You may eat all your favorite foods and desserts in moderation.

Eating Yourself Thin is about a lifestyle change. Changes where you begin to examine the amount of calories you burn in daily activities and the amount of calories you intake/eat daily.

As I examined my Current Eating Habits I ate six times each day. For every Meal there was the Snack before the next Meal and a Snack before bed. Plus I was hungry often during the day and if I woke up at night I would get a Snack.

.

Eating Yourself Thin

Talking to my physician about why I was hungry all the time. I was informed that this hunger was a side effect of the medicines that had been prescribed. The physician also informed me that one of the medications caused me not to process carbohydrates. Therefore I was not getting the nutrients needed for energy and the unburned carbohydrates were being stored as fat.

Well the greatest frustration was all the different diets I tried before and after this new knowledge. Each time I would lose 5 to 10 pounds. Only to gain the weight back over and over and over again.

Eating Yourself Thin

So realizing I was crazy trying the same thing over and over and expecting different results. I began to think about what one of my coaches had us do to maintain or lose weight to qualify for an event in a weight class. This was to synchronize the calories we burn daily with the calories in foods we eat daily.

So thinking about how much older I am now. I perform nowhere near the number of calorie burning activities I did in my teens.

This birthed the Eating Yourself Thin Strategy. "Eating Yourself Thin" is NOT a Diet and Exercising is Not Required.

Eating Yourself Thin

The strategy synchronizes the Calories We Burn Daily with the Calories in Foods We Eat Daily. To eliminate the excess calories not burned each day from being stored in the body. This allows you maintain or reduce your weight slowly having a long lasting effect.

I started at 235 pounds and I am now 187 pounds that is 48 pounds in about 2 years. My goal is 175 pounds, my doctors says its 170 pounds. I informed him that his charts were incorrect. This method is slow, you will have times of fast and slow weight release, be patient do not give up hope. It is a lifestyle change strategy not a diet plan.

Eating Yourself Thin

The nice thing about the Eating Yourself Thin Strategy is you don't get weight return whiplash when you stop.
I know because I like to eat every bake good in site at all the Holidays, cookouts, picnics, family reunions and secret emergency runs to the bakery. You may gain a pound or two but you just start using the Strategy again to return to the path of Eating Yourself Thin.

There are no special foods to buy, no classes to attend and no monthly fees. Not even an exercise plan because you match you intake calories to the calories you burn doing your normal daily activities. You can do additional activities to burn more calories.

Major components are prayer, drinking water (about two 20oz. bottles a day), reducing stress, getting proper sleep and positive affirmations.

Eating Yourself Thin

Positive Affirmations are essential you must encourage yourself. Others may not notice your progress as you do. Clothes fit better, you feel better yet people around may still say those unkind things. I believe they think they can shame you into taking action. NO amount of explaining can help most of them, you must encourage yourself. You know the hard work you are doing.

Just the other day I had someone say something really negative about my weight. In the pass I may have retaliated but today I just ignored them I know where I was and where I am now in my releasing weight process. Often I agree with people then they don't know what to say.

I am proud of my efforts mentally, emotionally and physically. I may not be where I desire to be but thank God I am getting better every day.

Eating Yourself Thin

Visualize your new self. I had suits that I could not even zip up the pants or button the coats. Yet I would not give them away because I had faith I would fit these suits again. Now I can get in most of those suits and I have suits and belts that are too big. Visualize your new self!

One of the greatest stress reducers I have found is "No Negative Conversations, No Displays of Anger"

What do you mean "No Negative Conversations, No Displays of Anger" we all get upset sometimes? Yes we all get upset and angry at times but it's our behavior afterwards that often does the most damage. Our behavior sometimes causes damage that is unrepairable.

We can control our behavior when upset or angry. We do it all the time at work and in situations where we want to impress or honor someone.

Eating Yourself Thin

In these instances we find a way to express ourselves that is non-offensive and non-threatening.

Why because we value these things and people, wanting to maintain a good relationship with them so we can continue to benefit from our association. We Respect these Relationships.

Well there is no one that we should respect, esteem, show admiration to MORE than our spouse and family.

No Negative Conversations, No Displays of Anger is a demonstration of LOVE.

Our commitment to No Negative Conversations, No Displays of Anger causes us to seek ways to telling the truth in love or with love.

Eating Yourself Thin

To find a way to express ourselves to our spouse and family that is non-offensive and non-threatening.

It shows we understand that other than God our peace, joy, comfort and security from the outside world begins with our spouse and family.

While also laying the ground work of respect for treating each other and how you treat all people.

No Negative Conversations, No Displays of Anger is a strong and powerful demonstration of LOVE.

This Love for Self transcends being moved by external irritations to achieving a peace that reduces our stress.

Stress that could lead to comfort food eating as a method to relax.

Eating Yourself Thin

Now back to examining my Current Eating Habits

Eating 6 times a day my Calorie Intake was 3000 to 3500 calories per day. While my daily activities only burned 1000 to 1800 calories per day. I was mentally stressed even more after this wonderful discovery.

But I needed to press forward because for my appearance, weight and health made me not feel like doing anything.

MY START CALORIES INTAKE – BURNED CHART

6 Meal a Day average

500 calories per meal = 3000

Calories Burned Daily = 1277

Calories Not Burned Daily Stored as Fat = 1723

Eating Yourself Thin

So I started small I stopped eating "HONEY BUNS" 480 calories each. Next candy bars 240 calories part of my work break routine. (NO HONEY BUNS AND CANDY BARS = 720 less calories per day) Slowly over the first year I was able to cut my intake down to about 2100 calories per day and now around 1900 calories per day.

Note: Your experience may be different. My first 30 pounds were hard but this last 18 pounds was much harder because those food commercials started looking so good. Yes I got some of that food to eat!

.

Eating Yourself Thin

One of the major issues I encountered was cravings for a special food I had remover for my normal eating habits. Like ice cream, cookies, cake, donuts or some other treat I loved. What I found, I would try to substitute healthy items for it but it would not satisfy the craving. So I would eat this and that and still end up eating that treat I wanted in the beginning. Wherefore if you have this issue it is better to eat that TREAT than to eat all other healthy food and end up eating the TREAT ALSO.

.

Eating Yourself Thin

<u>The Strategy</u>

1] Matching your intake of food to the amount of calories you anticipate burning each day.

2] Understanding your Current Eating Habits

3] Identifying and acknowledging foods you know you should not eat or eat less of.

4] Research any medical conditions or medications that may affect your body's Metabolism and digestion of food. This can affect weight loss or gain.

5] Using the <u>Calories We Burn Daily</u> charts to write out the number of calories you burn each day in your daily activities.

6] Using the <u>Food</u> charts provided to create your own weekly menu

    A] Identify number of calories you burn each day for 1 week

    B] Create a menu for 1 week that will reflect your intake being closer to what you burn each week.

Calories We Burn Daily

Calories burned in 30 minutes for people of three different weights

The table below lists the calories burned by doing dozens of activities listed by category (such as gym activities, sports activities, home repair, etc.) for 30 minutes. Activities are listed from least to most calories burned based on body weight. If you are above the maximum body weight as I was 235 lbs. use the 185 lbs. level.

	125 pound person	155 pound person	185 pound person
Weight Lifting: general	90	112	133
Aerobics: water	120	149	178
Stretching, Hatha Yoga	120	149	178
Calisthenics: moderate	135	167	200
Riders: general (ie., HealthRider)	150	186	222
Aerobics: low impact	165	205	244
Stair Step Machine: general	180	223	266
Teaching aerobics	180	223	266

Calories We Burn Daily

	180	223	266
Weight Lifting: vigorous	180	223	266
Aerobics, Step: low impact	210	260	311
Aerobics: high impact	210	260	311
Bicycling, Stationery: moderate	210	260	311
Rowing, Stationery: moderate	210	260	311
Calisthenics: vigorous	240	298	355
Circuit Training: general	240	298	355
Rowing, Stationery: vigorous	255	316	377
Elliptical Trainer: general	270	335	400
Ski Machine: general	285	353	422
Aerobics, Step: high impact	300	372	444
Bicycling, Stationery: vigorous	315	391	466
Training and Sport Activities			
Billiards	75	93	111
Bowling	90	112	133
Dancing: slow, waltz, foxtrot	90	112	133

Calories We Burn Daily

Frisbee	90	112	133
Volleyball: non-competitive, general play	90	112	133
Water Volleyball	90	112	133
Archery: non-hunting	105	130	155
Golf: using cart	105	130	155
Hang Gliding	105	130	155
Curling	120	149	178
Gymnastics: general	120	149	178
Horseback Riding: general	120	149	178
Tai Chi	120	149	178
Volleyball: competitive, gymnasium play	120	149	178
Walk: 3.5 mph (17 min/mi)	120	149	178
Badminton: general	135	167	200
Walk: 4 mph (15 min/mi)	135	167	200
Kayaking	150	186	222
Skateboarding	150	186	222

Calories We Burn Daily

Snorkeling	150	186	222
Softball: general play	150	186	222
Walk: 4.5 mph (13 min/mi)	150	186	222
Whitewater: rafting, kayaking	150	186	222
Dancing: disco, ballroom, square	165	205	244
Golf: carrying clubs	165	205	244
Dancing: Fast, ballet, twist	180	223	266
Hiking: cross-country	180	223	266
Skiing: downhill	180	223	266
Swimming: general	180	223	266
Walk/Jog: jog <10 min.	180	223	266
Water Skiing	180	223	266
Wrestling	180	223	266
Race Walking	195	242	289
Ice Skating: general	210	260	311

Calories We Burn Daily

Activity			
Racquetball: casual, general	210	260	311
Rollerblade Skating	210	260	311
Scuba or skin diving	210	260	311
Sledding, luge, toboggan	210	260	311
Soccer: general	210	260	311
Tennis: general	210	260	311
Basketball: playing a game	240	298	355
Bicycling: 12-13.9 mph	240	298	355
Football: touch, flag, general	240	298	355
Hockey: field & ice	240	298	355
Rock Climbing: rappelling	240	298	355
Running: 5 mph (12 min/mile)	240	298	355
Running: pushing wheelchair, marathon wheeling	240	298	355
Skiing: cross-country	240	298	355
Snow Shoeing	240	298	355

Calories We Burn Daily

Volleyball: beach	240	298	355
Bicycling: BMX or mountain	255	316	377
Boxing: sparring	270	335	400
Football: competitive	270	335	400
Orienteering	270	335	400
Running: 5.2 mph (11.5 min/mile)	270	335	400
Running: cross-country	270	335	400
Bicycling: 14-15.9 mph	300	372	444
Martial Arts: judo, karate, kickbox	300	372	444
Racquetball: competitive	300	372	444
Rope Jumping	300	372	444
Running: 6 mph (10 min/mile)	300	372	444
Swimming: breaststroke	300	372	444
Swimming: laps, vigorous	300	372	444
Swimming: treading, vigorous	300	372	444
Water Polo	300	372	444
Rock Climbing: ascending	330	409	488

Calories We Burn Daily

Running: 6.7 mph (9 min/mile)	330	409	488
Swimming: butterfly	330	409	488
Swimming: crawl	330	409	488
Bicycling: 16-19 mph	360	446	533
Handball: general	360	446	533
Running: 7.5 mph (8 min/mile)	375	465	555
Running: 8.6 mph (7 min/mile)	435	539	644
Bicycling: > 20 mph	495	614	733
Running: 10 mph (6 min/mile)	495	614	733
Outdoor Activities			
Planting seedlings, shrubs	120	149	178
Raking Lawn	120	149	178
Sacking grass or leaves	120	149	178
Gardening: general	135	167	200
Mowing Lawn: push, power	135	167	200
Operate Snow Blower: walking	135	167	200

Calories We Burn Daily

Gardening: weeding	139	172	205
Carrying & stacking wood	150	186	222
Digging, spading dirt	150	186	222
Laying sod / crushed rock	150	186	222
Mowing Lawn: push, hand	165	205	244
Chopping & splitting wood	180	223	266
Shoveling Snow: by hand	180	223	266
Home & Daily Life Activities			
Sleeping	19	23	28
Watching TV	23	28	33
Reading: sitting	34	42	50
Standing in line	38	47	56
Cooking	75	93	111
Child-care: bathing, feeding, etc.	105	130	155
Food Shopping: with cart	105	130	155

Calories We Burn Daily

	105	130	155
Moving: unpacking	105	130	155
Playing w/kids: moderate effort	120	149	178
Heavy Cleaning: wash car, windows	135	167	200
Child games: hop-scotch, jacks, etc.	150	186	222
Playing w/kids: vigorous effort	150	186	222
Moving: household furniture	180	223	266
Moving: carrying boxes	210	260	311
Home Repair			
Auto Repair	90	112	133
Wiring and Plumbing	90	112	133
Carpentry: refinish furniture	135	167	200
Lay or remove carpet/tile	135	167	200
Paint, paper, remodel: inside	135	167	200
Cleaning rain gutters	150	186	222

Calories We Burn Daily

Masseur, standing	120	149	178
Construction, general	165	205	244
Coal Mining	180	223	266
Horse Grooming	180	223	266
Masonry	210	260	311
Forestry, general	240	298	355
Heavy Tools, not power	240	298	355
Steel Mill: general	240	298	355
Firefighting	360	446	533

(This table was first printed in the July 2004 issue of the Harvard Heart Letter. For more information or to order, please go to http://www.health.harvard.edu/heart.)

Calories in Foods

MILK & DAIRY	Portion Size	Per 100g (3.5 oz)
Cheese average	110 cals (25g)	440 cals
Cottage cheese	49 cals (49g)	98 cals
Cream cheese	200 cals (47g)	428 cals
Eggs (1 average size)	90 cals (60g)	150 cals
Ice cream	200 cals (111g)	180 cals
Milk whole	175 cals (250ml/half pint)	70 cals
Milk semi-skimmed	125 cals (250ml/half pint)	50 cals
Milk skimmed	95 cals (250ml/half pint)	38 cals
Trifle with cream	290 cals (1 trifle)	190 cals
Yogurt natural	90 cals (1 small pot)	60 cals
Yogurt reduced fat	70 cals (1 small pot)	45 cals
BREADS & CEREALS	Portion Size	Per 100g (3.5 oz)
Bagel	140 cals (45g)	310 cals
Bread white (thick slice)	96 cals (1 slice 40g)	240 cals
Bread wholemeal (thick slice)	88 cals (1 slice 40g)	220 cals
Noodles (boiled)	175 cals (250g)	70 cals
Pasta (normal boiled)	330 cals (300g)	110 cals
Porridge oats (with water	193 cals (350g)	55 cals
Potatoes (boiled)	210 cals (300g)	70 cals
Rice (white boiled)	420 cals (300g)	140 cals
MEATS & FISH	Portion Size	Per 100g (3.5 oz)
Bacon average fried	250 cals (2 rashers)	500 cals
Beef (roast)	300 cals (107g)	280 cals
Chicken	220 cals (110g)	200 cals

Calories in Foods

MEATS & FISH	Portion Size	Per 100g (3.5 oz)
Ham	6 cals (2.5g)	240 cals
Lamb (roast)	300 cals (100g)	300 cals
Lunch meat	300 cals (75g)	400 cals
Prawns	180 cals (180g)	100 cals
Pork	320 cals (110g)	290 cals
Salmon fresh	220 cals (122g)	180 cals
Sausage pork fried	250 cals (78g)	320 cals
Trout fresh	200 cals (167g)	120 cals
Turkey	200 cals (125g)	160 cals
FRUITS & VEGETABLES	Portion Size	Per 100g (3.5 oz)
Apple	44 cals (100g)	44 cals
Banana	107 cals (165g)	65 cals
Broccoli	27 cals (84g)	32 cals
Cucumber	3 calories (30g)	10 calories
Grapes	55 calories (89g)	62 cals
Lettuce	4 cals (27g)	15 cals
Peas	210 cals (142g)	148 cals
Spinach	8 cals (100g)	8 cals
Strawberries	10 cals (33g)	30 cals

http://www.mypyramid.gov
http://nutrition.answers.com

Fast Food Drinks

In 1955, the standard "large" fountain drink cup at McDonalds was <u>seven ounces</u>. Today, the *smallest* cup — a child's size — is 12 ounces, and the adult cups range in size from 16 to 30 ounces. Head to other fast food joints, and you can find servings as large as 64 ounces. (For those counting at home, that's more than *double* the capacity of the average <u>human stomach</u>!) That means you can order up a vessel of soda that'll cost you up to 700 calories a pop.

To make matters worse, soft drinks aren't the only beverages served in mega-sized containers: Additive-packed smoothies, fat-filled shakes, and sugar-loaded coffees also come in these gigantic sizes. And with the longer ingredient lists come hundreds of additional calories.

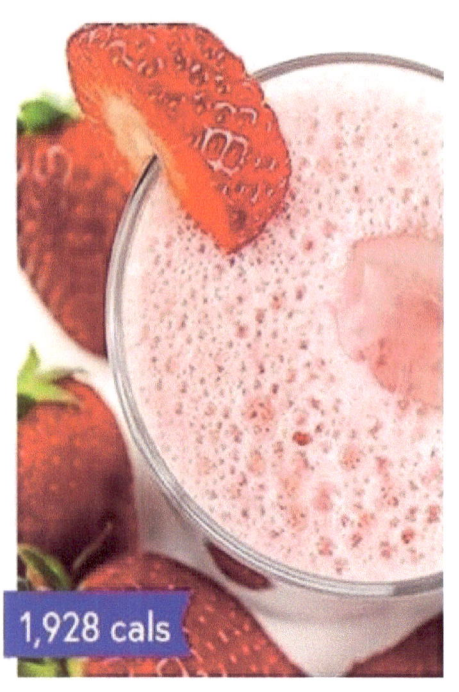

1,928 cals

1. [Smoothie King The Hulk Strawberry]

Nutrition Facts: A large (40 oz) contains 1,928 calories, 64 g fat (26 g saturated fat), 250 g sugar and 50 g protein.

2. [Dunkin' Donuts Frozen Mocha Coffee Coolatta]

Nutrition Facts: A large (32 oz) contains 990 calories, 47 g fat (29 g saturated fat), 125 g sugar and 8 g protein.

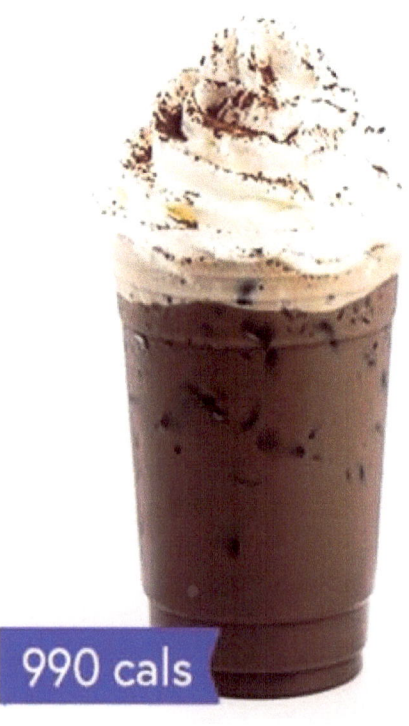

990 cals

3. Jamba Juice Peanut Butter Moo'd Shake

Nutrition Facts: A large (28 oz) contains 980 calories, 29 g fat (6 g saturated fat), 131 g sugar and 26 g protein.

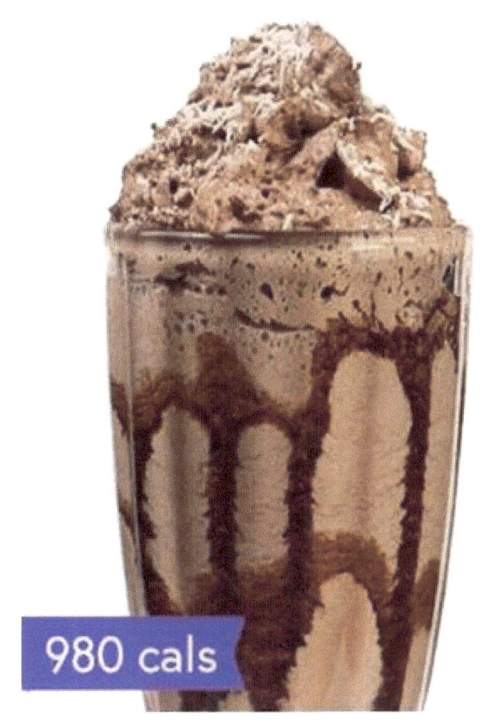

980 cals

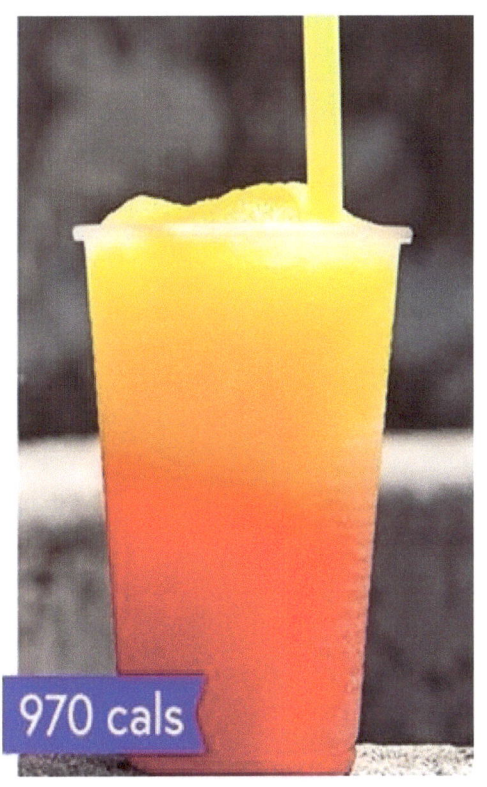

970 cals

4. Sonic Grape Slushie with NERDS Candy

Nutrition Facts: A "Route 44" size (44 oz) contains 970 calories, 0 g fat, 247 g sugar and 0 g protein.

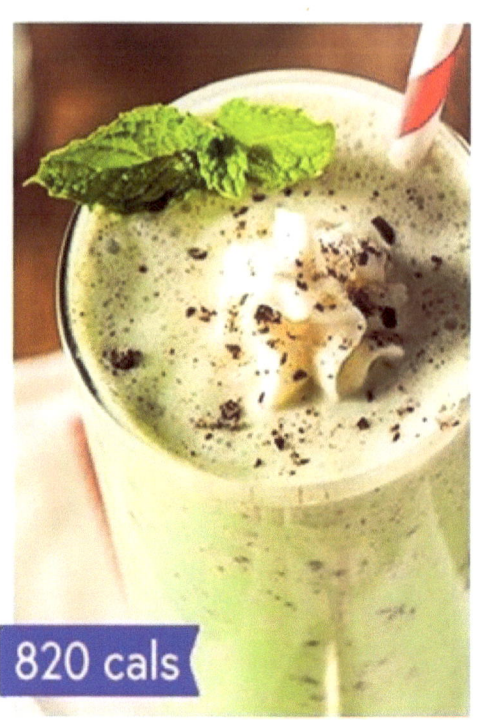

820 cals

5. McDonald's Shamrock Shake

Nutrition Facts: A large (22 oz) contains 820 calories, 23 g fat (15 g saturated fat), 115 g sugar and 18 g protein.

6. Starbucks Peppermint White Chocolate Mocha

Nutrition Facts: A venti (20 oz) contains 680 calories, 26 g fat, 94 g sugar and 19 g protein.

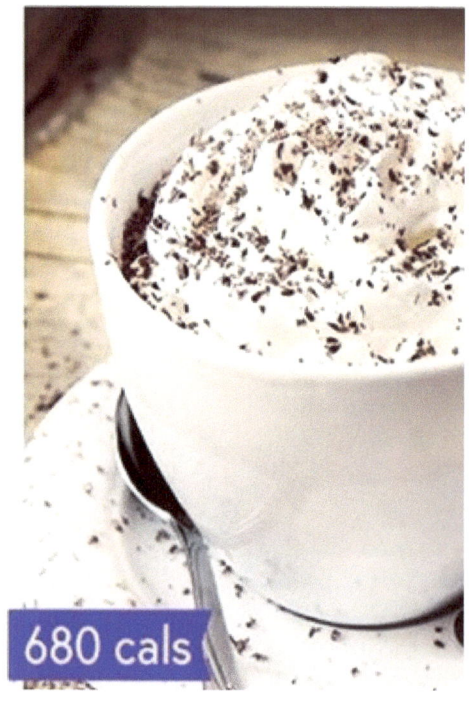

680 cals

7. Wendy's Chocolate Frosty

Nutrition Facts: A large (20 oz) contains 580 calories, 15 g fat (10 g saturated fat), 80 g sugar and 16 g protein.

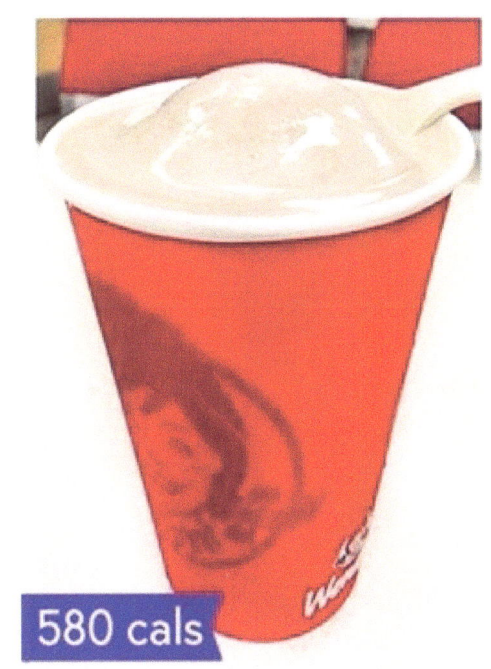

580 cals

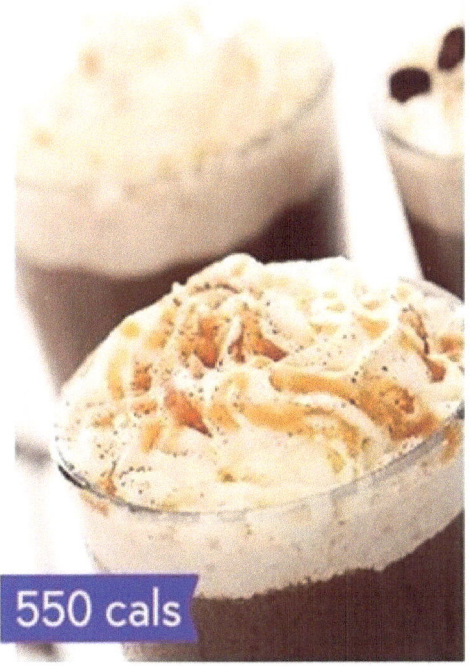

550 cals

8. Starbucks Salted Caramel Mocha Frappuccino

Nutrition Facts: A large (24 oz) contains 550 calories, 18 g fat (11 g saturated fat), 90 g sugar and 7 g protein.

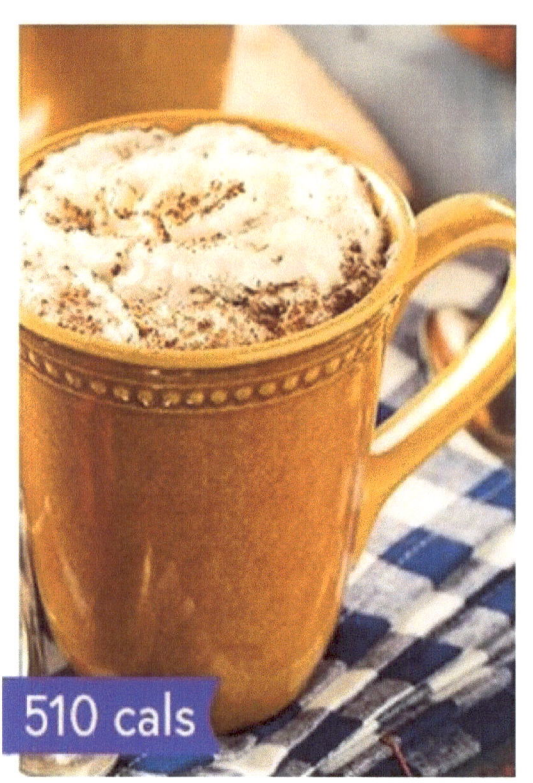

510 cals

9. Starbucks Pumpkin Spice Latte

Nutrition Facts: A large (20 oz) contains 510 calories, 20 g fat (12 g saturated fat), 62 g sugar and 18 g protein.

10. Dunkin' Donuts Iced Pumpkin Mocha Latte

Nutrition Facts: A large (32 oz) contains 470 calories, 13 g fat (7 g saturated fat), 71 g sugar and 14 g protein.

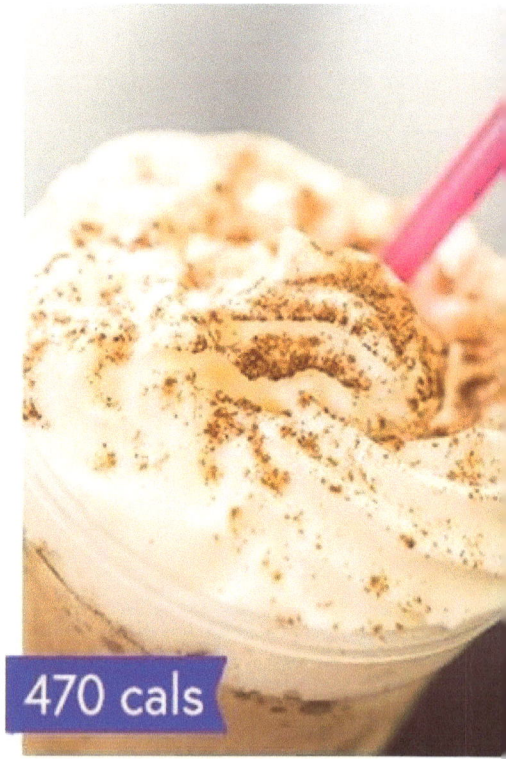

470 cals

11. Seven-Eleven Fanta Wild Cherry Slurpee

Nutrition Facts: A Big Gulp size (32 oz) contains 263 calories, 0 g fat, 72 g sugar and 0 g protein.

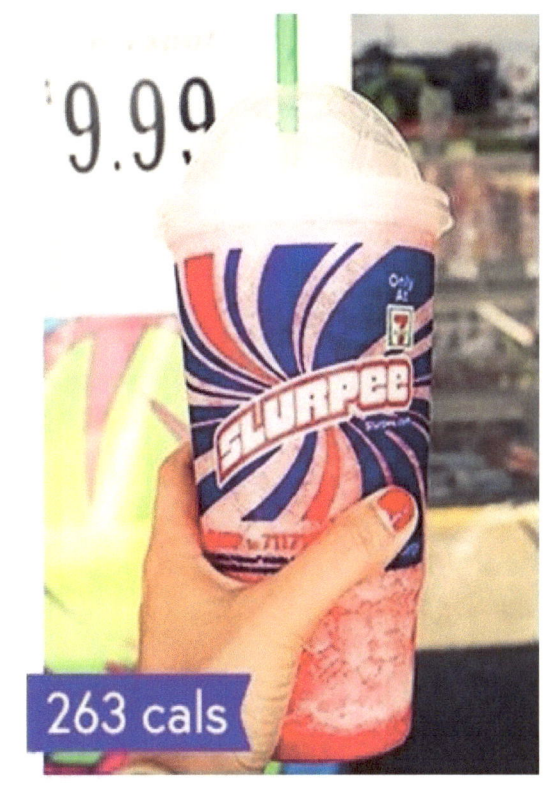

263 cals

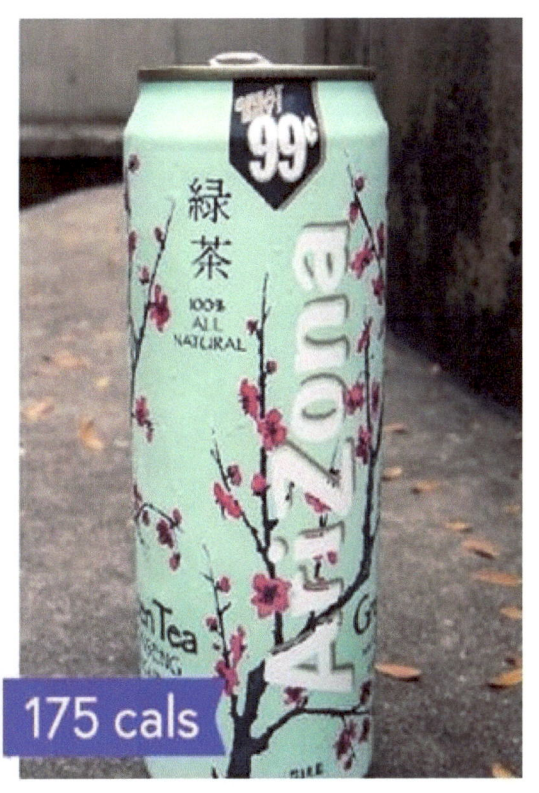

175 cals

12. Arizona Green Iced Tea with Ginseng and Honey

Nutrition Facts: A tall can (20 oz) contains 175 calories, 0 g fat, 42.5 g sugar and 0 g protein.

Appendix

Exhibits

Current Eating Habits

Calories Burned Daily

Current Eating Habits

Monday	Tuesday	Wednesday	Thursday	Friday	Saturday	Sunday
Breakfast	Breakfast	Breakfast	Breakfast	Breakfast	Breakfast	Breakfast
Snack	Snack	Snack	Snack	Snack	Snack	Snack
Lunch	Lunch	Lunch	Lunch	Lunch	Lunch	Lunch
Snack	Snack	Snack	Snack	Snack	Snack	Snack
Dinner	Dinner	Dinner	Dinner	Dinner	Dinner	Dinner
Snack	Snack	Snack	Snack	Snack	Snack	Snack

Example Chart

Calories Burned Daily

Activities	Calories	Activities	Calories	Activities	Calories	Sub-Total
						Calories
Computer Work	61	Sleeping	28	Stair Step Machine: general	266	**355**
Light Office Work	67	Watching TV	33	Child-care: bathing, feeding, etc.	155	**255**
Sitting in Meetings	72	Reading: sitting	50	Food Shopping	155	**344**
Desk Work	78	Standing in line	56			**134**
Sitting in Class	78	Cooking	111			**189**
				Total	Calories	**1,277**

Example Chart

FORGIVE

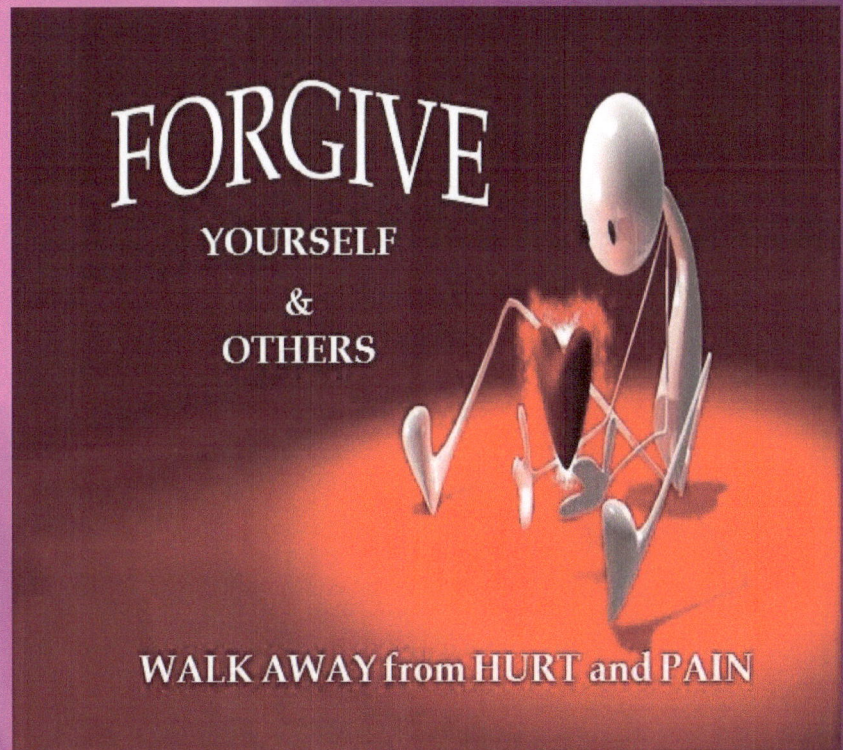

FORGIVE
YOURSELF
&
OTHERS

WALK AWAY from HURT and PAIN

WILLIAM EDWARD TURNER

In 40 Days

Marriage Re-Newal

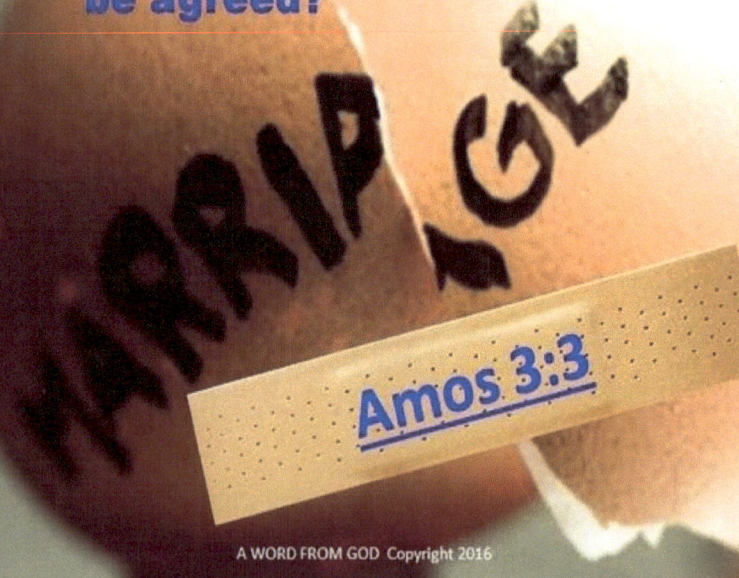

Can two walk together, except they be agreed?

Amos 3:3

A WORD FROM GOD Copyright 2016

WILLIAM EDWARD TURNER

Marriage Coach – Certified Biblical Counselor

The Relationship Exam

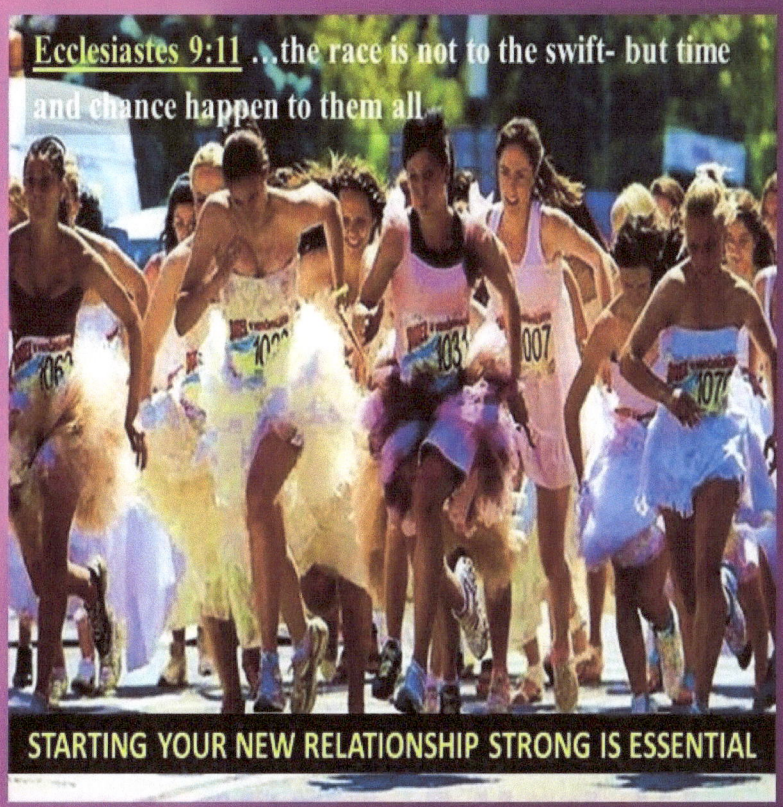

Ecclesiastes 9:11 ...the race is not to the swift- but time and chance happen to them all

STARTING YOUR NEW RELATIONSHIP STRONG IS ESSENTIAL

William Edward Turner

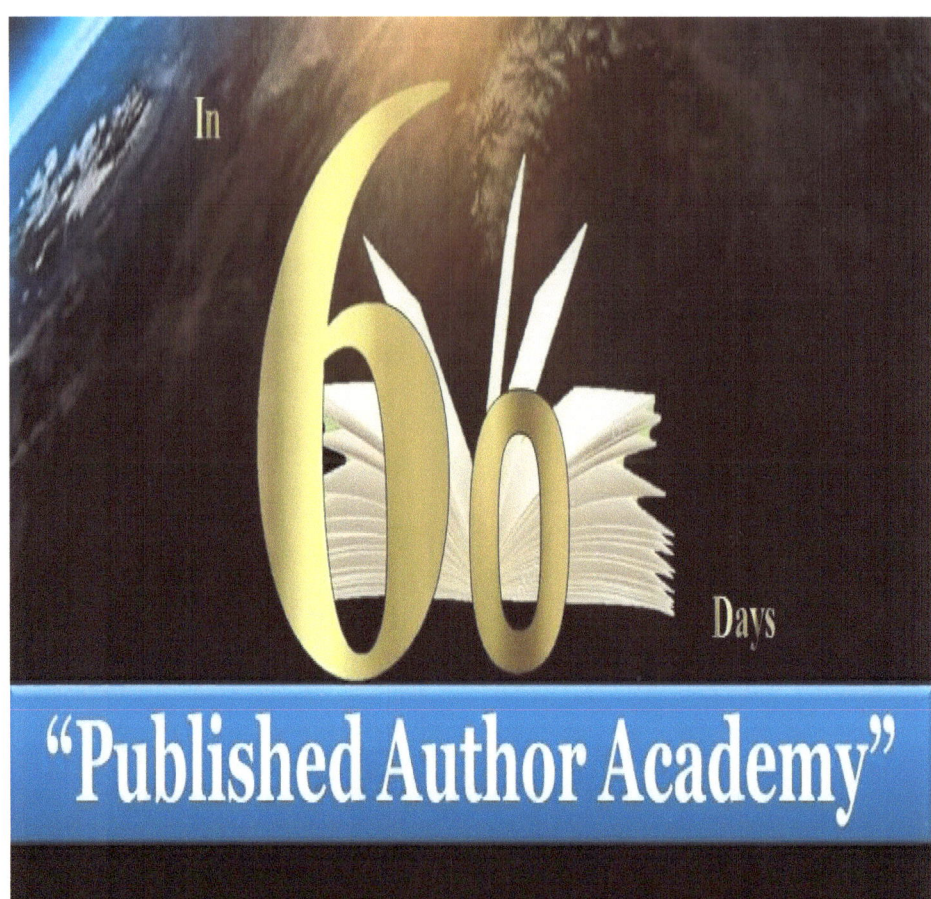

In 60 Days

"Published Author Academy"

336-706-0090

wmedward@outlook.com

www.ingramcontent.com/pod-product-compliance
Lightning Source LLC
Chambersburg PA
CBHW050840290526
45792CB00001B/470